Crystal Healing for Modern Life

Published 2024
Published by Spiral Moon Circle Publishing,
an imprint of Spiral Moon Media Group, Troy, MI, USA
https://publishing.spiralmoon.net
https://spiralmoonmedia.com
ISBN: 978-0-9914926-2-6

Crystal Healing For Modern Life

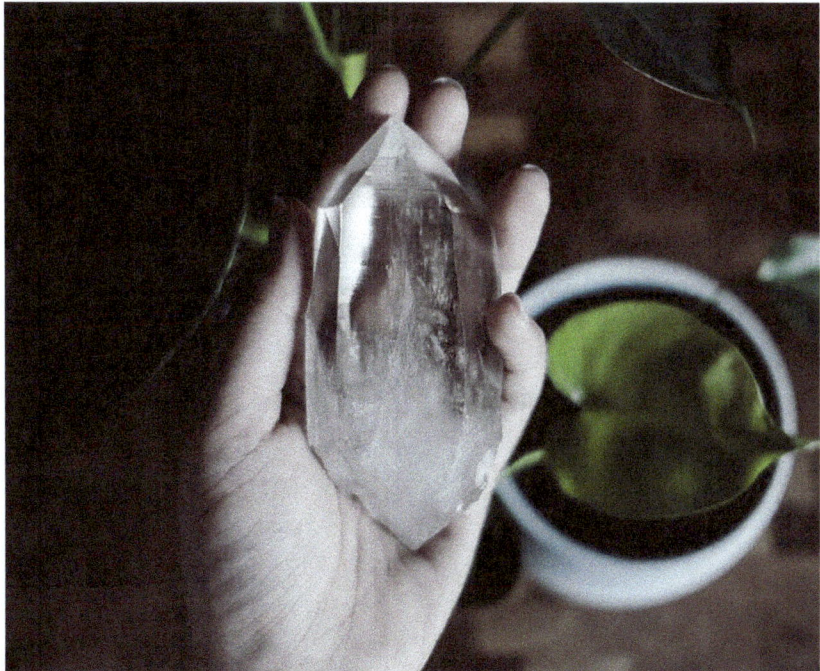

Foreword

Crystal therapy or crystal healing is a type of vibrational medicine. Crystal therapy typically involves the application of crystals or gemstones to aid in the healing of one's body or spirit. Gemstones hold spiritual and healing attributes that may be tapped into in a myriad of ways. Crystals can be carried or worn on the individual or placed in a location where their therapeutic vibrations may be felt by whosoever is nearby. Healers likewise, place stones on their clients' reclined bodies to equilibrate the chakras and aura.

Chapter 1: What's Behind Crystal Healing

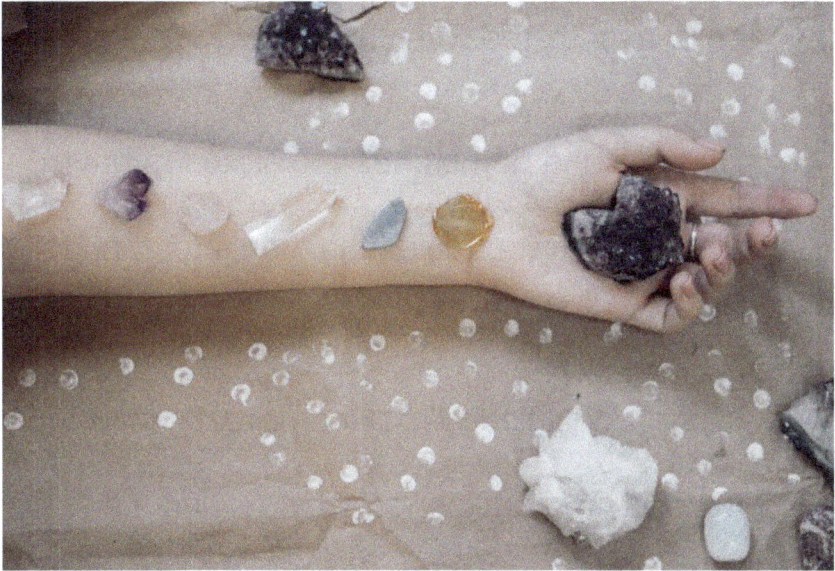

An Introduction

Crystal healing is a type of healing that utilizes crystals or gemstones. The crystals are primarily placed on particular areas of the body called "Chakras." Chakra is a Hindu term implying *spiritual energy*. According to the teachings, there are 7 general energy centers in the body, and each one features a different color associated with it.

Crystals and gemstones are stated to have vibrational frequencies that can interconnect an individual with earth's energy fields. The crystal is utilized to expand or realign human psychic or cosmic energy by guiding the vibrational energy.

Some crystal healers lay the same color crystals as the color of the chakras on the individual to heighten the flow of energy. Many other crystal healers generally prefer to work with clear quartz, because of its shape and color. Crystals can guide the flow of energy to a certain part of the body and in turn, bring

balance to their overall energy and well being.

To maintain the crystal, it's laid in salt water or

covered with table salt. Sustaining the crystal

helps keeps them clean from "environmental

unbalance". Just as any important item of ours

needs upkeep and care, your crystals need to

be recharged periodically to keep them

functioning at their highest level.

Ultimately, crystals can be used to pull out

damaged energy from an individual. Driving

out the defective spiritual energy eases

physical ailments. Crystals are utilized for

physical, mental, emotional and spiritual

healing. Not only can individuals visit crystal healers, in a few places, professional nurses are trained to utilize crystals for their patients as well. In addition, crystals may be worn, placed next to a bed as one sleeps, or placed around a warm bath.

Practically from the very dawn of humankind, people have been utilizing amulets, magical stones, talismans and gems for all manners of healing and protection. Many people might be surprised upon learning that there were crystal healers practicing over 10,000 years ago! Although historically practiced in mostly Eastern cultures, this powerful knowledge is finally making its way to the western world. As the technological world creeps closer and closer to our society we can only assume that the search for healing will increase as the years go on. Crystals may play a vital role in this "awakening" as more and more people look for new modalities of healing.

Chapter 2: Ramping Up Your Energy

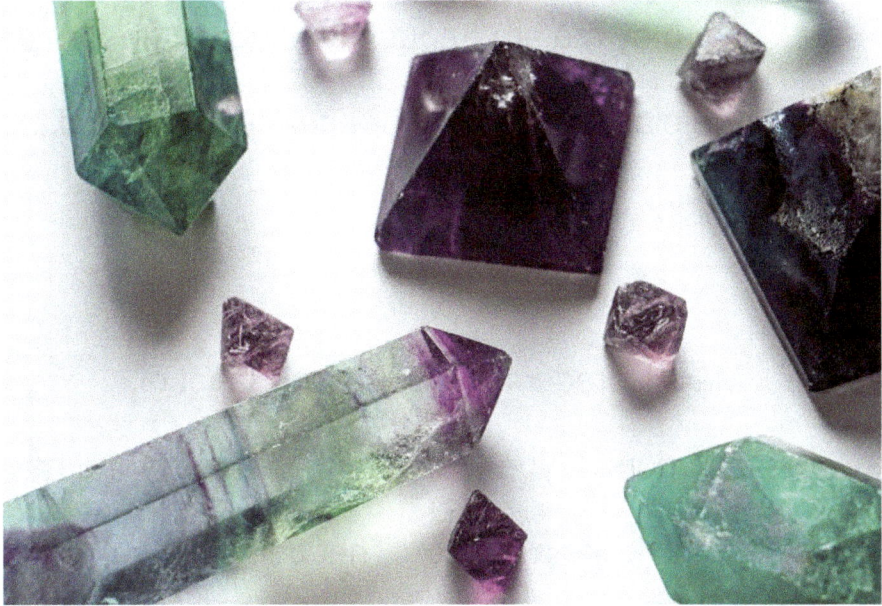

Crystals for Power

Below is a list of crystals that may help you

and provide that much-needed supercharge of

energy. Broadly speaking, if faced with

tiredness, pick out stones that are connected

with the component of Fire. This component is energy personified. You'll discover that stones ruled by fire are frequently ruled by the Sun or the planet Mars, and are nearly always red in color.

Mars is frequently called the Planet of Warriors. If you wish to fight fatigue, you'll have to think like a warrior. That being stated, the crystals in that category are Ruby, Garnet, Red Jasper, and Amber. And as fatigue might bring with it rounds of depression and/or insomnia, Amethyst and Green Aventurine are useful crystals to heal these ailments.

Ruby is a crimson crystal that's ruled by the component of Fire and the planet Mars. This potent energizer step-ups blood flow, heighten stamina, and presents you with renewed energy. Utilize it on the sacral or root chakra. Raw, rough rubies are much less expensive and are perfect for this sort of healing. Reload rubies utilizing a soft cloth to wipe them down and put them on a windowsill at nighttime to be charged up by the stars.

Garnet is a burgundy-red stone that's ruled by Fire and the planet Mars as well. Put on the root chakra, it may improve circulation, as well as expand that sense of vitality you might be missing. This warming crystal may be worn or carried in a pocket (as with all of these crystals) and it may be recharged even on a mirky night.

Red Jasper is the "Warrior Rock". This red rock is, like Ruby and Garnet, ruled by Fire and Mars. It's indispensable if you have to step-up stamina, heighten circulation and want to give an awesome boost of energy to the system. It's affiliated with the root chakra and may be recharged by passing it through a red standard candle flame.

Amber, the fossilized leftovers of ancient tree resin, is affiliated with Fire and the Sun. This fiery, golden-orange stone reloads your energy levels by arousing a more favorable attitude. If your emotions are running rampant due to emotional overcharge, lay amber on the solar plexus or sacral chakra to counterbalance those emotional tensions. It may be reloaded by placing it on a sunny windowsill.

Amethyst is a quieting stone for those enduring fatigue ascribable to emotional overload. This purplish crystal is ruled by the component of Air and the planet Jupiter. It's thought of as an awesome healing stone for emotional weariness, insomnia and headaches. It likewise balances blood glucose levels and has been recognized to recharge other stones. Put it on your brow chakra or beneath your pillow at night. Naturally, it may be worn or carried. Recharge amethyst by putting it in moonlight, as this stone shouldn't be placed in direct Sunlight.

Aventurine, while green, is a marvelous crystal for clearing off negativity, increasing optimism and affecting a more favorable outlook. It's a more gentle stimulating stone, but may still encourage a regenerated zest for life. It's an earth stone and is ruled by Mercury. Aventurine is utilized on the heart chakra to quiet panic-attacks and nervousness affiliated with emotional fatigue. It may be recharged by placing it in amongst the leaves of a plant during the day.

If you've ever experienced a lack of energy or fatigue after lunch this sort of afternoon energy slump may be alleviated with your crystals, rather than having to grab a caffeinated drink or sugary snack. Crystals that are going to hike up that afternoon slouch are ruby, amber, and jasper. Ruby and Amber are reloading stones and will jumpstart your system. A different one to try is aventurine, which will add a little optimism to the mix.

What if you're having difficulty sleeping? You're so worn out from your everyday life and stress, you feel as if you could sleep for a week, but your mind won't switch off. Cup of

Chamomile Tea? Maybe. Some calming music and a little meditation? Go for it. Rose Quartz and Amethyst will likewise bring a more relaxing sleep if placed beneath your pillow. These are quieting stones that will greatly help those with overtaxed brains and bouts of insomnia. A different stone to help you relax is blue lace agate that, if held in your hand, will help your entire body relax. The crystal Iolite can also help with insomnia along with headaches, eyestrain, and mental tension, by working to calm those overtaxed nerves.

So, whether you're a long-distance runner or simply running through the stress of day-after-day, I hope one or more of these crystals will help you to battle your fatigue and bring you serenity and energy.

Elements, Planets, and Crystals

At this point, a few of you might be wondering why the elements and planets are named in many of the crystal descriptions. Every element – Earth, Air, Fire and Water – and every planet – from the Sun to Pluto – corresponds to assorted energies, emotions, attributes, colors, and so forth.

Fire, for instance, is affiliated with the color red and is utilized for physical strength, staying power, protection, energy and bravery. Water is blue and is utilized for healing, relaxation, rest, and psychic Powers.

Earth is regulated by green and is utilized for grounding, peace, constancy, fertility, cash and gardening/agriculture. Air is yellow and is the component of communication, travel and all matters regarding the intellect.

Mentioned here were Mars, the Sun, Jupiter and Mercury. Mars is for bravery, passion, protection and strength and is governed likewise by red. The Sun deals with physical power, protection, healing and success and its color is golden or yellow. Jupiter is for meditation, spirituality, success, and psychic cognizance and its color is purple. Mercury regulates communication, wiseness, self-reformation, study, and travel, and its color is yellow.

Chapter 3: All About Amethyst

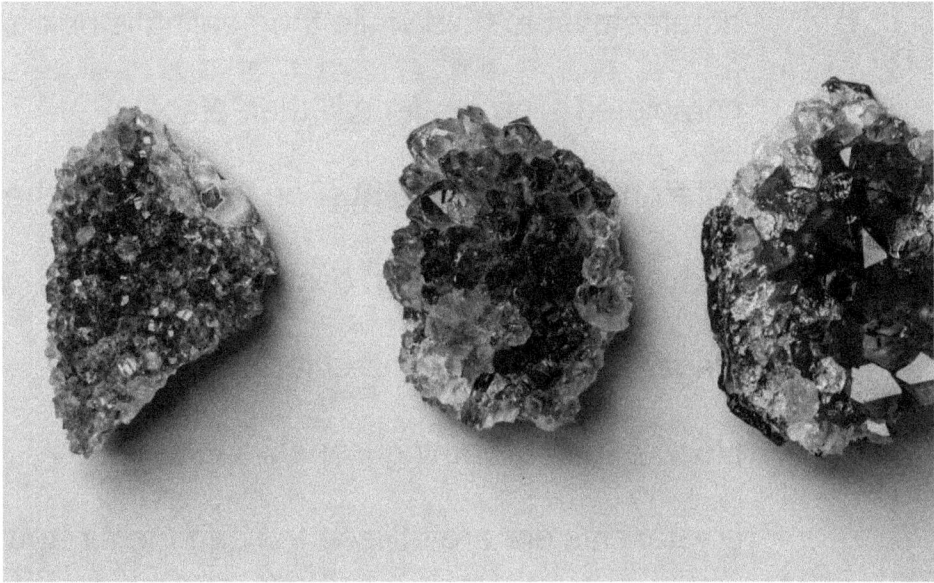

What This Stone Is Used For

Amethyst is a gemstone frequently worn by

healers, as it has the ability to center energy. A

healer will commonly wear various pieces of

jewelry with amethysts set in silver, particularly

an amethyst necklace.

Oftentimes, the person being healed will have an amethyst to hold while the healing is being completed. The healer will then place a different piece of amethyst on the areas of the body that need healing, commonly the heart or lungs. Amethyst is utilized for issues in the blood and in breathing issues. Amethyst crystal clusters are utilized to keep the air and vitality in the home clean and favorable.

Place Amethyst clusters, points or tumbled stones in moonlight to help everybody in the home to feel less agitated. Utilizing an amethyst as a meditation center will expand positive spiritual feelings. Amethyst helps defeat fears and cravings. It likewise helps alleviate headaches.

Hold an amethyst stone in each hand when meditating. It's an excellent stone to use while meditating because it can aid in more intense visualizations. Another thing you can do is place a couple of amethyst stones around the rooms where tempers might frequently be riled. It's a stone of peace and helps bestow love and happiness to all who utilize it.

An Amethyst stone makes an awesome gift for anybody that works as a psychic or those that show psychic powers, as it helps increase all forms of psychic abilities.

If you endure migraines, here's a simple crystal healing curative that has been known to help. Lie down and shut your eyes. Put an amethyst stone on your brow and attempt to relax and let the gemstones do their work.

Muscle and joint traumas, such as sprains, can be healed quicker by putting an amethyst stone inside an elastic bandage that is wrapped around the wounded area.

To assist with breathing issues, along with any medications from the doctor, put an amethyst on the chest, between the lungs. Dependent on the severity of the illness, you may be able to actually tape a stone in place with a band aid and slumber with it in place.

To make an amethyst stone elixir, put one or more amethysts into a clear glass jar full of water. Let the water sit outside in the moonlight for the whole night. The closer to the full moon, the better. Use this amethyst water to help clear up blemishes and soften the skin. You may wash with it or utilize it as an ingredient in any clays or masks you might apply.

You may also make an Amethyst Stone elixir and utilize it to bathe the parts of the body that are undergoing circulatory issues. It can step-up circulation in both the physical body and the etheric.

If you discover yourself having issues sleeping at night and spend more time tossing and turning than really sleeping, place an amethyst stone beneath your pillow to help with insomnia.

To expand the number of dreams that you have and to help you recall your dreams when you awaken, utilize an elastic hair band as a head band around your forehead. Slip an amethyst stone beneath the band as it is known to help facilitate dreaming.

Bury a little amethyst stone at every entrance to your house to guard against thieves. A cheap strand of amethyst chips works perfectly for this. Don't forget to bury a little beneath every window, as well as the doors. If you have a window that's far away from a place where you can bury the stones, such as a window above a cement patio or porch, simply put a tumbled stone or crystal on the windowpane.

Utilize the same technique above to protect against thieves and to keep evil from your household. This will also help keep all who wish you or your loved ones harm, from attempting to come into your home.

To commune with your Spirit Guide or Higher Self, discover a peaceful time and place where you won't be interrupted. Carry an amethyst stone in each hand. Take a couple of deep breaths, shut your eyes feel the powers come from the amethyst. Invite your guide to come forward and talk with you. This helps you attune with your higher self.

With the hectic world moving so quick around us, we frequently find ourselves strained beyond the capacity the human body was designed to endure. Spend a couple of minutes absorbing the power of amethyst crystals to help mend the nervous system and

feel more at peace.

Chapter 4: Apatite

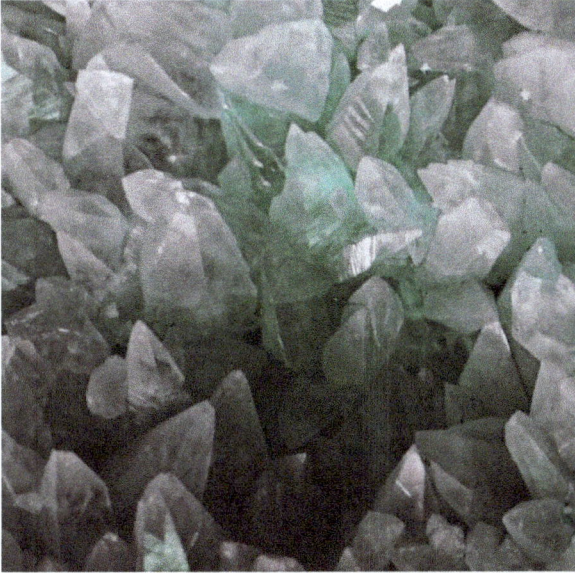

Psychic Development And More

It's frequently been stated, before you can change something, you must accept it as it is. An apatite gemstone crystal is a multi-talented gemstone assisting us attune to our inner selves and take on inner and outer healing, communication, and balancing. Apatite is the perfect gemstone for utilization on any of the chakras as it can both perk up under activity and calm down over activity and clear congestion in any of the chakras.

Apatite gemstone crystals aid in the development of psychic powers and can help you attune your mind, heart and soul to the spiritual forces that run throughout the universe.

To expand your power to receive visions of the future, meditate with an apatite gemstone leaning against your third eye chakra (somewhat above and between the eyebrows). Blue or purple colored apatite gems work best for this.

Apatite gemstone helps bones to mend faster and stronger. It aids in your body's absorption of calcium from the foods you consume, which helps to keep bones and teeth strong.

To help ease arthritis pain, wrap the involved joint in an elastic bandage allowing it to hold one or more stones against the impacted joint. The apatite gemstone may help heal the painful sensation and heal the joint quicker.

Produce an elixir by placing one or more apatite gemstones in a glass container of water and let it sit outside overnight, preferable under a full moon. This elixir may be drunk to help strengthen bones and heal and prevent joint pain.

To help lower hypertension, wear an apatite gemstone so it hangs just above the heart. Wearing one on a chain works well, but if you are unable to do this, simply pin a stone to the interior of your shirt.

If you realize you have the tendency to let your emotions rule instead of logic, particularly in emergency type situations, apatite gemstone crystals may be your resolution. This

gemstone will let calm prevail presenting you

the time and power to let logic rule in the

Situation.

Wear one or more apatite crystals while

executing any kind of creative work. It helps

you to link up with your creative center and

produce spectacular works.

Does shyness or doubt forbid you from

enjoying yourself at parties or in additional

social situations? An apatite gemstone may

provide you

the confidence to feel comfortable in social settings and provide you the feeling of security you require to shine at your best.

Do you require a little extra motivation to get the job finished? A gold or red apatite gemstone held during meditation may help you keep your mind centered on the subject at hand presenting you the desire to continue working till completion.

Chapter 5: Green Serpentine

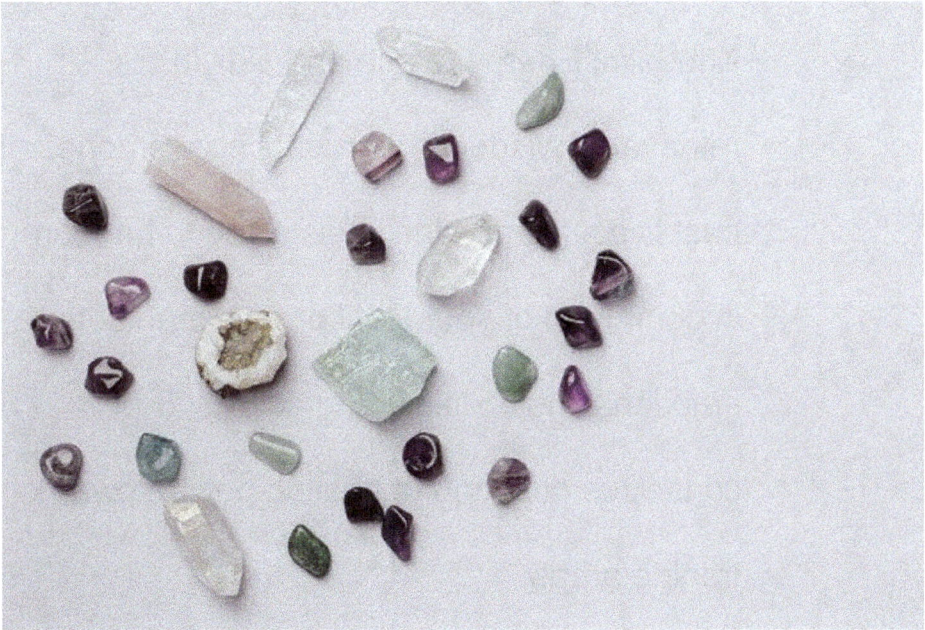

Detox For The Body

Serpentine is an earthling stone that helps

meditation and spiritual exploration. It clears

up the chakras and energizes the crown

chakra, opens psychic powers and helps us

comprehend the spiritual basis of life.

This stone opens fresh pathways for the Kundalini Energy to rise and aids in the retrieval of wisdom and regaining memories of past lives. Serpentine assists you to be more in command of your life, corrects mental and emotional instabilities, and assists the conscious direction of healing power towards trouble areas.

Physically, Serpentine mineral is exceedingly cleansing and detoxifying for the body and blood to assure longevity. It does away with parasites, aids calcium and magnesium absorption, and treats hypoglycemia and diabetes.

Light-Green Serpentine is a gentle, tender-natured stone that can help you receive contact with a source of angelic guidance. It helps to integrate the past, present, and future, making it an awesome stone for past-life exploration.

This stone encourages compassion and forgiveness for yourself and for what you have experienced. Holding this stone leads you into the healing regions that exist in the between-lives state. This way, the healing that wasn't undertaken after a former life ended may now be accomplished.

This stone heals instabilities from past lives and clears up emotional baggage from old relationships. If placed on the throat, it helps with speaking of the past and resolves issues carried forward into the here and now. This stone is awesome to utilize when you want to confront anybody from your past, as it brings in a gentle touch to the meeting.

Physically, light green serpentine is awesome for pain relief, particularly menstrual and muscular aches and pains.

Chapter 6: What Turquoise Can Do

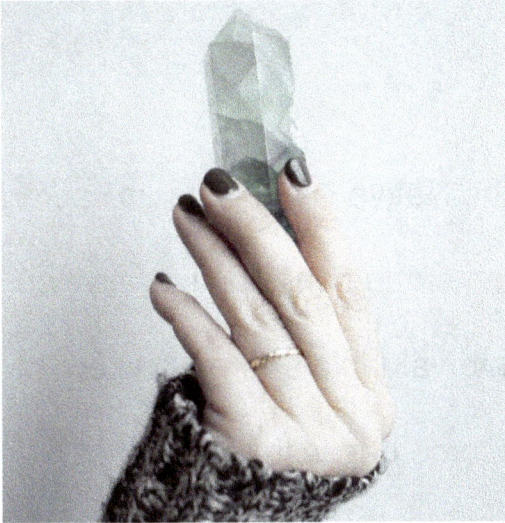

A Sacred Healing Stone

Turquoise is the healing stone that attunes our physical selves to the greatest realms. It helps us to better comprehend ourselves and to bring our thoughts and emotions under control . You've but to stop and listen, be quiet, and be prepared to hear the truth about whom and what you are. Simply then will you find your full power.

Respected by the Native Americans as sacred, the turquoise gemstone soaks up negativity, transmuting it into valuable energy. It likewise helps you to become one with the cosmos. The real turquoise meaning comes from the heart and the soul of the individual utilizing it.

The list of turquoise gem healing attributes is long and wide-ranging and the assortments of turquoise crystal shapes, sizes, and colors that may be utilized are as wide-ranging as the individuals that utilize Them.

Worn any place on the body, a turquoise gem healing stone will protect and bless the wearer. It's considered a hallowed stone in some cultures, personifying a gift from the gods.

A strand of turquoise gemstone crystal beads worn around the neck soaks up all negativity from the body and brain and helps you formulate your own innate powers. You are able to align your chakras by laying a turquoise stone on each of the chakra points for 3 to 5 minutes while the gem executes its work. If you don't have seven turquoise stones, it might take a bit longer, however, laying a single stone on one chakra at one time for the same three to five minutes will still align your chakras for the best level of power.

A strand of turquoise beads utilized as a bracelet, necklace or even an anklet will help detoxify the body from alcoholic beverages, pollution, poison and radiation. The thought is to wear a circle of beads around one area of the body so as the blood flows back and forth through the area, the turquoise may purify it.

Anybody that has issues with their lungs, throat, or from asthma, may hang a turquoise gemstone from a cord or chain so it hangs immediately over the area causing the issue. This helps the gem energies get as close as possible to the trouble area and start the

healing work.

Those suffering from depressive disorder may

sleep with a turquoise gemstone to help lift

depression.

Add a couple of turquoise crystals to a

container of water and let it sit outside where

the moon may shine on it overnight and the

sun may shine on it over the next day. That

evening, pour the turquoise water into a warm

bath, step in, sit down and let the healing

energies work on your body. This same

healing elixir may be utilized to soak a

sprained or pulled muscle, strengthen the

immune system so you may fight off viruses and infections, and assist in healing damaged or cut tissues. For headaches, soak a cloth in the elixir and put on your brow till the pain disappears.

Chapter 7: Quartz

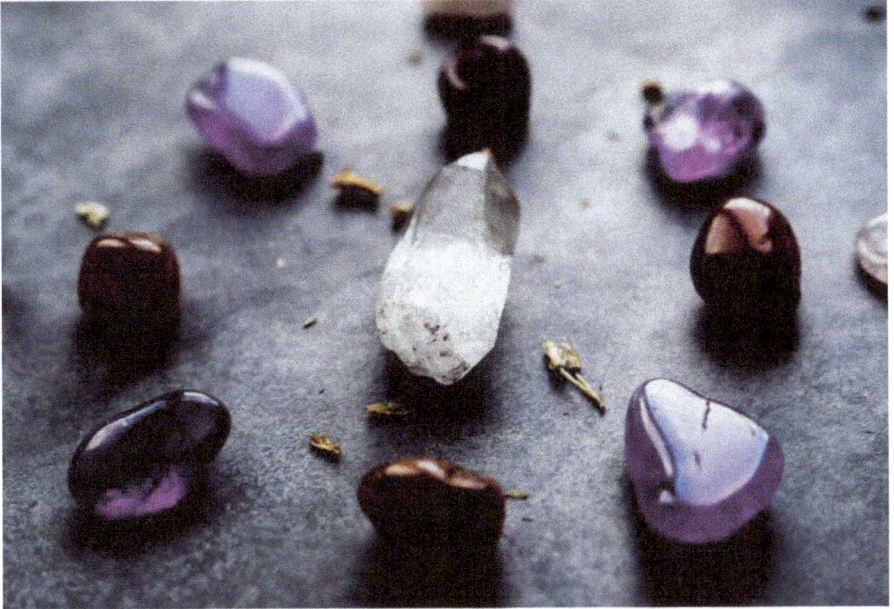

A Crystal Healing Essential

When it comes to the range of crystals utilized in spiritual healing nothing stands higher than quartz. The healing energies of quartz have long been recognized. Since the time of the fabled Atlantis no stone has been more revered for its crystal healing attributes than quartz. To the shaman and metaphysical healer, quartz is the quintessential curative stone. Quartz crystals possess all of the attributes the practitioners of Crystal Healing look for.

Even science realizes the unparalleled and astonishing abilities of quartz crystals. The crystalline structure of quartz carries electricity and radio frequencies. It's why Quartz is utilized in radios and additional electronic devices. And why scientists are experimenting with quartz and additional crystals as sources of possibly unlimited alternative energy.

There are a lot of different types of quartz crystals, and each one has their own unique healing powers and impact different parts of the Body. For instance, rose quartz is utilized by crystal healers for headaches, the handling of heart issues, and kidney disease. Clear quartz is utilized to draw out pain, bring back clarity of consciousness, and to broadly amplify all curative energies. However, all quartz crystals have the power to realign the vibrations of the body, restoring balance. That's what makes quartz crystals so efficient in healing. Most disease issues, but particularly mental disorders and neurological issues may be linked to some sort of "chemical" or "neurotransmitter" instability. The influence of quartz crystals may help mend these imbalances.

The electro-magnetic attributes of quartz are mostly due to the base of its crystalline anatomical structure being made up of silica. Silica is a natural occurring glass. Silica is detected in some level in nearly every healing crystal, chakra stone, or ritualistic gem. Silica, likewise, shares its chemical and molecular construction with silicon, known for its electro-magnetic attributes.

Chapter 8: Bloodstone

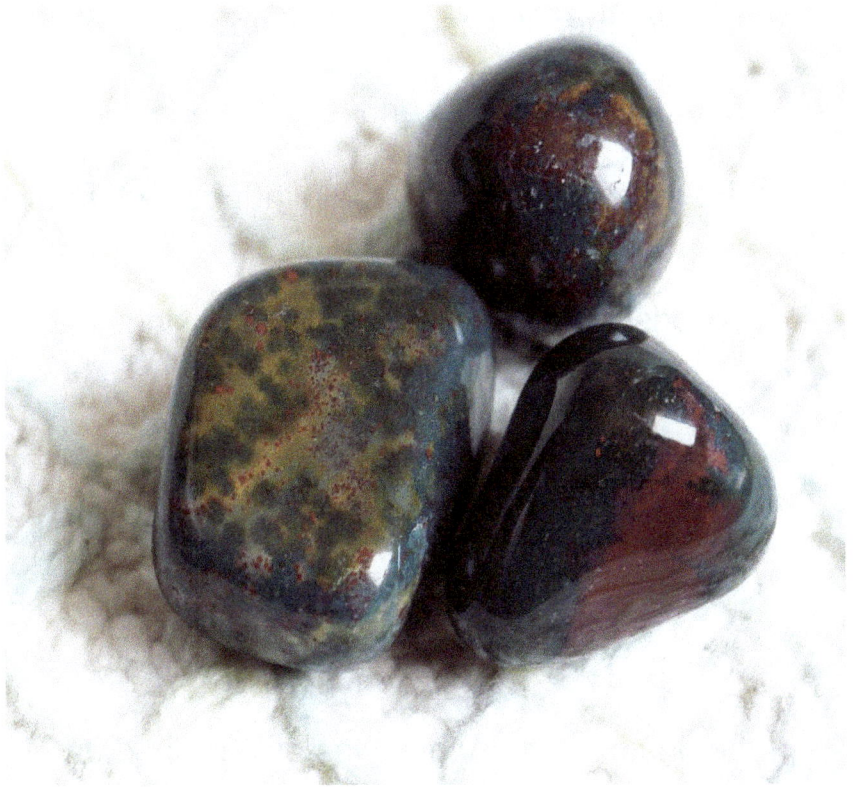

A Stone for Creativity, Healing, and Bravery

Formerly, bloodstone crystals were called heliotrope. The word heliotrope is compiled of the Greek word for 'the sun', *helios* and the Greek word for 'to turn', *trepein*. The historical uses of the stones were to induce changes in the weather. It was thought if you place a bloodstone in water and let the stone suck up the rays of the sun, it would induce a storm.

Bloodstone advances creative thinking, self-expression, and artistry. In the Middle Ages, bloodstone was ground into a powder, blended with honey and eggs and given to patients to heal tumors. A paste made of mashed bloodstone and honey was also rubbed on cuts to stop bleeding.

As a healing stone, a bloodstone is utilized by healers to help with any sort of blood disorders. This includes but isn't limited to anemia, circulatory issues and Lupus.

Wearing or carrying a bloodstone helps to strengthen the immune system, clean toxins from the liver and kidney and purify the bone marrow. This makes it an awesome stone for women as it helps to alleviate both menstrual and menopausal symptoms.

To help cure snakebite, affix a bloodstone to draw the poison out of the bite. Notice, this was an ancient utilization of the stone. You may do this while on the way to acquire medical help, but do not do this rather than seeking medical attention.

The ancient Babylonians utilized engraved bloodstone in divinations. They utilized the way the assorted spots of red looked to tap into their psychic powers, producing an effect similar to a vision by following the array of the spots.

To purge your mind, body and soul, on the night of the full moon, find a place outdoors where you may lay under the moons light. Put a stone on your forehead as you lay down and relax. Visualize the moon's power entering your body, filling it with perfect white light. As your body fills, see all the negativism, illness and tension leaving your body, and sinking into the ground under you.

Ancient Egyptians utilized bloodstone magic to assist them in battles. They utilized magical empowered stones as amulets for the warriors to expand their personal strength.

Athletes may utilize a bloodstone amulet to help expand their strength and speed. Wear or carry a stone and visualize its power entering your body and inducing your muscles to become stronger or Faster.

This same magic may be utilized by anybody in need of bravery to get through a situation. Simply envision the powers entering the body and presenting you with the strength that you require.

To turn "invisible" to your foes, wear or carry a bloodstone and visualize a cloak of power emanating from the stone and enfolding around you, making you unseeable to those you don't want to be seen by.

If you know of somebody that tends to be a bit too self-centered, give them a gift of a bloodstone. It helps them to see how matters affect not just them, but other people around them or even the whole world.

Hold a bloodstone in your hands with meditations designed to help you connect with your preceding lives. Once you've entered the meditative state, turn your thoughts backward

to a time before your birth and let the images

guide you to sights of your prior lives.

Keep one or more bloodstones on your desk or

worktable to help expand your business and

riches. Even people that don't run their own

business may benefit by letting the stone draw

in additional sources of money into their lives.

Chapter 9: Choosing The Right Crystals

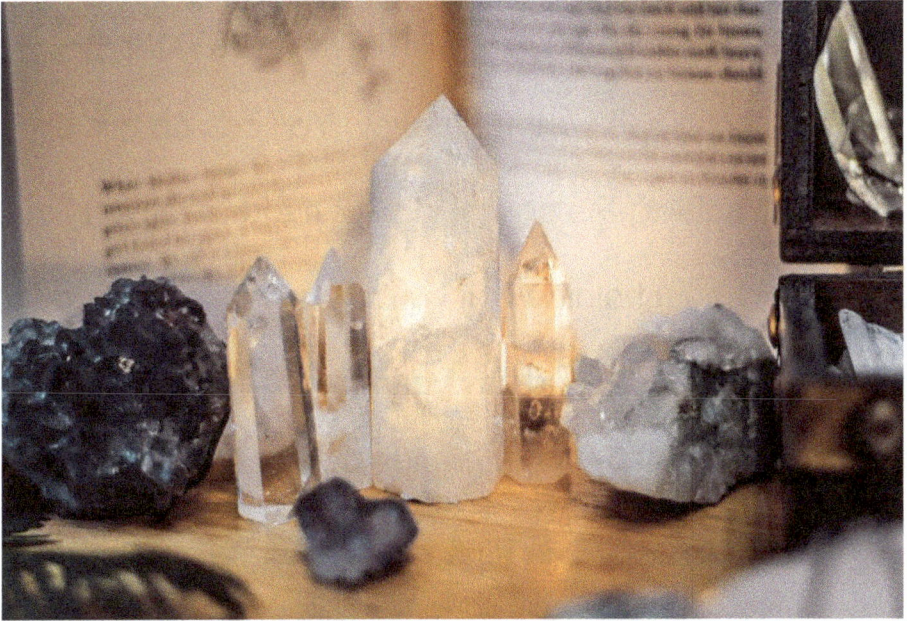

How to Choose a Crystal

Here is an easy procedure to identify which

crystal will work best for your specific goal.

First, seek a few crystal assortments that appear to support your goal. Then select a particular crystal that provides a vibrational match to your frequency. You can do this by holding the crystal in your hand or thinking about holding it (if you're purchasing online for instance) and say your purpose. For example, "I want to feel more at peace." Always say the purpose in an affirmative sentence, do not say something like, "I wish to quit feeling angry". Affirmative sentences allow the flow of energy (which is what you require), while damaging sentences trigger resistors.

Shut your eyes while you say your purpose out loud. If you're more in-tuned with your emotions, seek a positive feeling from your stone (lightness, tingly, happy, excitement are great emotions to look for).

If you're more in-tuned with your body, you might be able to utilize muscle testing. You can try this out by balancing yourself upright, letting your body "hover" and then falling in the way your body wishes. If you fall frontwards, it means you have a great match. If you fall backwards, you don't. There are a lot of different ways to utilize muscle testing for this intent, this is just one example.

Once you've discovered the right crystal for you, make a conscious effort to let yourself be open to its influence. To interact with the tangible world, we frequently have to shut down our receptivity to outside influences. That may lead to a generalized shutdown where all influences are blocked. Be aware that you may discover yourself inadvertently fighting the crystal's influence.

One last thing you can do to facilitate the healing vibrations of your crystal is to place your crystal close to a water fountain. Don't place them in the water, as the mineral deposits may damage them. But any spot near a fountain will do. This lets the really powerful chi of the water propagate the vibrational frequency of the crystal throughout your space.

Conclusion

When you look for the help of a crystal, you're enlisting a potent ally to raise your vibrational frequency. Regardless of what the crystal is utilized for, its desired effect is always to increase your vibrational frequency. We frequently crave particular crystals because we have a great "vibrational match" with them. This vibrational match implies that proximity to this crystal elevates our vibrational frequency, therefore, making us feel great.

Choosing a crystal for a particular purpose is an awesome way to help yourself without having to commit much energy to it. The proximity of the crystal is perpetually affecting your own frequency, maneuvering you upward towards your goal.

In conclusion, I hope this book was helpful and that you now have the information you need to begin your own crystal healing journey. Just remember to trust your intuition and be open to new healing vibrations and you are sure to find the power, healing, and support you are searching for.

www.ingramcontent.com/pod-product-compliance
Lightning Source LLC
LaVergne TN
LVHW021135080426
835509LV00010B/1361